Finish Rich -
The Dentist Retirement Bible

FREE RESOURCES FOR YOU

Here is a chance for you to dig deeper into details surrounding a transition plan for you.

There are several resources FREE to you including...

- A Free Practice Appraisal valued over $5,000
- A Free Cash Flow Analysis of Your Practice
- A resource center with hundreds of articles written specifically for doctors in need of a transition strategy
- A free transition plan designed specifically for your needs

Just Visit: www.aftco.net

Click on the "Selling A Practice" tab at the top of the page for FREE resources

PREFACE

This book is written to help dentists who are uncertain about how or when to begin the process of slowing down and/or retiring or even choosing a different path for their life. Tim & Chad are extremely knowledgeable in providing transition strategies, as they have over <u>30 years</u> of combined experience in the dental world, both as analysts and as practice owners.

Their journey began with an affiliation with the largest and oldest dental practice transition company in the country. AFTCO started in 1968 and began by brokering practices in the traditional strategy of practice sales. Since their formation in 1968, AFTCO's team has completed over **$2.3 billion** worth of sales in well over 10,000 transitions.

The initial approach by AFTCO shifted in a few short years from only being brokers working for a commission to a careful examination of the needs and goals of the seller. This became a crucial difference between the traditional broker and a real strategist who finds a candidate who would fulfill the objectives of the seller. To do this, the needs and goals of a potential purchaser candidate must also be examined. Once an understanding of the needs and goals of both seller and buyer are understood, a higher practice value can be obtained for the seller and the purchaser receives greater value and typically becomes 50% - 100% more successful. This is what we call a win-win transition. Because of this win-win philosophy, once a buyer has been introduced to a

4

seller, it has an 80-90% successful closing rate, using this non-adversarial approach. This means more money for the seller and greater return for the purchaser.

Chad and Tim are an informed, experienced and impartial third-party who represent the interest of both parties involved in a practice transition. Our policy of this concept of dual representation assures both parties that we will be completing a fair and equitable win-win transition. Throughout the years our commitment of dual representation has enabled us to develop a reputation for professionalism, integrity and fairness, resulting in both parties receiving full value in the transition. We work *very* hard to create a win-win transition on *every* acquisition.

If you're the type of person that feels that every transaction is a zero-sum game where you must cut the legs out from the purchaser to get ahead, then this is not the book for you. But, if you are looking for a fair transition where you can hand pick the best candidate not only for you, but for your staff and patients, then this is the *best* book you will ever read on this topic.

Some Background Info

In 1995, Tim Wildung formed the group Family Dental by purchasing the first practice. By 1998, it had grown to 8 practices. Family Dental then merged with Dental One in late 1998 and together they grew to 55 practices by 2002. In 2002 alone, both Tim and Dental One acquired nearly 100 additional practices. Many of these were acquired to merge into their current practice facilities. This gave them the opportunity to hire numerous dentists, hygienists and staff members. Having done this, this gave them a much greater understanding of the dental business and what it felt like to be a practice owner. It also came with many successes and a few failures. They found that they learned as much or more from the failures than the successes. They often found themselves saying that they truly have done everything a dentist does except turn the hand-piece.

Using this acquired understanding and experience, Tim has helped many dentists figure out their goals and step out of feeling trapped in dentistry. Tim's goal is creating a path to achieve whatever the dentist wants in life, whether that means continuing to work with less stress, changing careers or just retiring to enjoy the fruits of their labors.

Chapter 1

Why So Many Dentists Fear Retirement

You weren't born a Dentist; you should not die a Dentist.
Alan F. Thornberg

Case Study:

Dr. A, a 74-year-old dentist in southern Arizona, was considering selling his practice and retiring. He had been considering doing this for over 15 years, and each time he would examine his financial condition with his financial advisor yet received the same answer every time: "*You must work another 5 years.*"

Dr. A had always spent 110% of what he earned. Even though he had been earning a net income of over $500,000 per year, he could not retire. His debts would take everything and he would be left with just social security to live on. His wife said, "you can do this" and he just continues to work and faces the inevitable-- he will die at the chair over a patient!

Dentists fear retirement. Many people view retirement as an opportunity to enjoy life without the hassles of business or employment. Dentists, on the other hand, fear retirement because it represents change. As we know, most people don't like change and would prefer to avoid it if possible. Dentists tend to feel that retirement means they have reached the end of their productive years and that they are now being "put out to pasture."

Many people believe that retirement is anything but unproductive. It represents an opportunity to focus on all those things in life that have been put off because of the pressures and responsibilities that accompany their "productive years." Dentists tend to think that retirement represents "throwing in the towel" before the "game" is over; it means admitting that they are mortal.

Putting off retirement is usually an attempt to avoid acknowledging one's mortality. The average dental practice is composed of patients who represent an average cross-section of society, or more accurately, a cross-section of the local community, with different social and economic backgrounds. Many patients lack the financial resources to approaching retirement with the sense of security and rewards that a dentist should expect to enjoy. Many retired patients are tired, burned out, of poor health or have little money to enjoy their "golden" years. Television becomes the way to pass the time and those retirees quickly become bored and restless. They fondly recall their "productive working years" forgetting about the stress that was so long associated with those memories.

Retirees need more care and see doctors more often than any other type of person, and they are accustomed to talking to as many individuals as possible about their problems. They often complain to their dentist (who happens to be a captive listener) about their inactivity, boredom, sickness and often financial woes. Some people will die shortly after retirement, and their family members believe the cause of death was retirement rather than the years of being overworked and overstressed. The advice frequently heard by dentists from their well-meaning patients is, "Avoid retiring, Doc!"

Thus, a dentist's perspective on retirement is greatly influenced by his patient base. He begins to associate retirement with inactivity, boredom and even death. As years go by, the doctor slowly starts to realize that he is approaching retirement age as the kids finish school and get married, he pays off his mortgage and he does not have the same responsibilities that he once had. He then begins to think about all those patients he has seen over the years. They retired, became sick, complained a lot and then they died. They did not enjoy retirement. Well, he is not going to fall into that trap!

This is where it becomes interesting. Some people might view this scenario and conclude that to enjoy retirement one should retire as early as possible while still healthy, and not put it off until his health is spent. Retire early, live longer and enjoy more healthy, happy and productive years. Take the time to pursue the things in life you've always wanted such as traveling the world, the theater, participating in sports and reading-- the activities that there was never time for before retirement.

Yes, this would seem to be a logical conclusion for most people. It is safe to say that this is the advice a dentist would give to his or her children if given an opportunity to advise them on this same matter. What do most dentists do instead? They practice until they die! Instead of retiring early and having a long, happy and healthy retirement as a reward for a lifetime of service to others, they let death become their final reward. Instead of time spent with their loved ones, instead of traveling and seeing the world, fishing, golf hunting...they work until they die.

Dentists do have options few others can afford. Most dentists do not have to practice until they die. Dentists can have a long, happy and productive retirement, and if they'd like, they can even sell their practice now, eliminate the responsibilities associated with ownership and continue to practice full or even part time. Dentists can phase into retirement years before they thought possible and live longer as a result. Correctly planned, dentists can have it all.

Dentists and "Procrastination"

You're getting older and you know that you need to make plans to do something with your dental practice, but you are not exactly sure what to do. You've been considering your retirement options, but you think, "Why hurry? I've got time on my side." Procrastination--the great common denominator for so many doctors. Why not put off until tomorrow what one does not have to do today (or next month, or next year)?

Procrastination is not an overt act; an overt act requires thought and action, which is just the opposite of procrastination. A good procrastinator must also be good at rationalizing inaction. As a matter of fact, procrastination and rationalization go hand in hand. Let's combine those two words and call it "procrastinalization."

A practice is one of the most valuable assets most doctors own. Putting off a decision for the transition of your practice can be one of the costliest "procrastinalizations" a doctor could ever make in his or her lifetime. As retirement approaches, the financial health of the doctor at the time of retirement will dictate the quality of life for the doctor and spouse for 5, 10 or even 50 years. No one knows how long he or she will continue to live or remain disability free. If you die or become disabled, you could lose 50% to 100% of the current value of your practice. If you are rich, then it's no problem. If you are not rich, however, "procrastinalization" can be a real issue.

Now, let's review a few common "procrastinalizations" and see if you have been using any of them:

1) "I know my practice is worth a lot of money if I can keep up the production, so what is the risk? What could happen to my practice? Tomorrow might not come, you say...no way. But, now that I think about it I will do something about my practice tomorrow."

2) "Retire? For what? I've got my health. I feel good. I've gone this far without doing anything. So, what's a few more months or years for that matter? Who knows, I may have five or even ten more good years left before I need to retire, so why worry!"

3) "I've got to work until I'm sixty-five! What's that you say? Did I turn sixty-five three years ago? Well then, I have to work until I'm seventy."

4) "No, I'm not going to die before I retire. Disability? I didn't think about that. I'll reflect on that tomorrow. It's not part of my retirement plan and probably won't even happen!"

5) "I have to keep practicing dentistry because I need a place for my wife to work!"

6) "I am not procrastinating. I'm a D.D.S., which stands for 'Deferred Decision Strategy'. I've used it often to formulate a plan for my future. It will work for me, you'll see. I am going to get it started next week."

How Can Retirement Work with Proper Planning?

Case Study:
Dr. B was nearing the age where he began to think about retiring and enjoying life. What would he do, how would he leave his patients and whether anyone else could care for them as he had for so many years. He decided to sell his practice, so a suitable purchasing dentist was found. Dr. A could reduce his work schedule to 1-2 days per week and work for the new owner. He found this very fulfilling because he could continue his relationship with favorite patients and have "Dr. New" see old Mrs. Jones who was always complaining that nothing was ever done well enough. This was great-- all of the joy of practicing and very little of the frustrations. If equipment broke down, Dr. A would inform "Dr. New" and take the rest of the day off. When Susie at the front desk got pregnant and quit, no worries, "Dr. New"

would be the one to deal with it. Dr. B felt like he could go on like this forever!

Dr. B purchased a motor home and began to travel with Mrs. B. This was a lot of fun and soon Dr. B did not miss the office any more. The patients loved "Dr. New", much to Dr. B's secret surprise. After about 3 years, Dr. B decided to completely retire. Dr. B had received enough for his practice to have a sizable nest egg, plus he had financed half of the sale so he had a monthly check coming in for the next 10 years. With his pension, social security and this monthly check, Dr. & Mrs. B could travel and enjoy life more than ever before without even touching the nest egg. After the 10 years had passed, the nest egg had grown enough that it more than replaced the monthly payments that were no longer coming in. Now at age 78 Dr. & Mrs. B are continuing to enjoy their "Golden Years" in true fashion.

If You Fail to Plan, You Plan to Fail

Benjamin Franklin supposedly once said:
"If you fail to plan, you are planning to fail."

Sir Winston Churchill is credited with another saying:
"Those who fail to learn from the past are doomed to repeat it."

Imagine if you could create the ideal scenario where you could get maximum value out of your practice at just the right time while continuing to do that which you most enjoy. Sell your practice at its peak and invest the proceeds into an investment that would produce passive income for the rest of your life. This takes planning and expertise to orchestrate an ideal transition into the next phase of your life.

You were not born a dentist and you should not die a dentist. If you identify at all with what has been written to this point, then you owe it to yourself and your family to begin your journey now. We have been working with dentists for over 28 years by helping them create and take advantage of the most beneficial way to make transitions. It has happened for literally hundreds of dentists across the country and can happen to you when you take the appropriate steps toward your ideal future.

Reach out to us to begin your journey.

At AFTCO, we help dentists/owners create a plan to achieve financial independence and retirement. It's never too early to begin creating a plan. In fact, our most successful dentists began working towards their retirement goals decades before actually retiring.

Discover how your retirement goals can be achieved by calling 480-634-4803 or visiting our website at www.aftco.net.

Chapter 2

<u>Determining Needs and Goals</u>

Setting goals is the first step in turning the invisible into the visible.
Tony Robbins

A Sad Story

Case Study:
A dentist died not too long ago. He had a growing practice in a desirable, suburban location. He died without a will (intestate) and without instructions for the disposal of his practice. Here is what happened:

The grieving widow contacted her husband's attorney and accountant. Neither individual had any idea how to sell a practice, nor were they aware of how much value a practice would lose by delaying the sale. They instructed the staff to forward all patient calls to another dentist in the same town while they tried to determine what to do next. This action considerably decreased the value of the practice, since most of those patients referred to another office would probably remain with that dentist out of convenience.

The weeks lead into months while the practice was appraised by the supply house (they were not interested in their potential customers buying the equipment from this practice). Potential purchasers were informed that the practice no longer had any value since it was closed for so long. The accountant and supply salesman listed all the supplies and counted every instrument, not knowing that this had little effect on the overall value of the practice. A practice's real worth is patient load, not the tangible assets.

Meanwhile, as time marched on, the practice value continued to decline. Three months from the time the dentist died, the attorney decided to accept bids for the practice. Where there had been a long list of potential buyers, there remained two interested parties, both of whom were looking for a "Good Deal." At the time the dentist died, there were buyers willing to pay $480,000 to $500,000 for his practice. Because of the delays, the final selling price was less than $200,000.

Retirement... When and How?

The dream of a lifetime...out with the old and in with the new...the "Golden Years" and a new chapter in life, etc., etc., etc. Sure, a new chapter that's exciting and means no office to go to every working day, heck, no more working days, period! A lifetime of running a dental practice can make you crazy and the prospects of having no patients to treat, no practice to manage, no staff to oversee sounds so good, but what comes next?

Retirement! Think of it as day after day of playing golf, or fishing, or traveling, or visiting family, etc., etc., etc. Well, ok, that might work for the first year or so, but then what do you do with all this free time after that? Well, you might try jigsaw puzzles, board games, cards or even (God forbid) shuffleboard! Retirement itself becomes a cliché. You need something to do to break the boredom.

Instead of welcoming every weekend break like you did when you were practicing dentistry, you now don't know what day of the week it is without looking at a calendar. At least when you were practicing dentistry you had something to feel good about and something else to complain about, which in a way made life more interesting. Now one day seems like every other day and boredom sets in, then another form of craziness takes over.

Ok, so maybe you aren't cut out for retirement. So maybe there is a need for another alternative to retiring and quitting dentistry, but what is it? Let's look at what needs to be taken into consideration as a dentist approaches his or her "Golden Years."

Rule number one for everyone. Secure the value of your dental practice, which, for many dentists represents one of the most valuable assets they have in their financial portfolio. This money can provide financial security and improve your quality of life during the next ten or twenty years or so. Too many dentists wait to sell their practice until they are ready to quit dentistry and often lose 50% to 100% of their practice value. Not securing the value of your practice is one of the costliest mistakes a dentist can make at a critical time of their life, so don't let that happen to you.

Now, the next consideration is whether you still enjoy clinical dentistry or not. If you do not enjoy clinical dentistry any longer, then, provided you have enough money set aside to retire in reasonable comfort, retirement is your chance to quit and get out of dentistry, which you should do. You've climbed the mountain, slain the dragon and now you can devote your time to all those other pursuits that you have been daydreaming about for years. There is no need to read more of this article, just make sure you get the full value for your practice and put it in a safe place because you will need that money to secure your financial future.

If you still enjoy clinical dentistry but are getting up there in years, then there are some options available to you besides quitting dentistry and retiring. We find that many dentists still enjoy the clinical side of dentistry, but that the stress they experience comes from the responsibilities of managing the dental practice. You never own a dental practice-- it owns you. As a practice owner, your choices are minimal at best. If you think not, then let's see you take a month off for a vacation, start working two or three days a week instead of the four or five you are now working or cut your office hours down to four hours a day. Is that enough proof? That's right; you can't do these things because you are responsible for the practice…you don't own it-- it owns you!

So, what would be the ideal situation for any dentist as he or she is approaching the "Golden Years"? The first objective would be to get paid now for the full value of your practice and use that money to provide additional future financial security. Every day you "own" your dental practice is another day that you are at risk for losing that practice value. If you became sick, disabled or die, your practice value would drop faster than the value of the Edsel after it was introduced by Ford back in the late fifties. Practices right now are at an all-time high (60% and up to 100% of a year's gross income in some areas) and taxes on the sale of a practice are at an all-time low. Delaying this important step can cost a lot of money to the average dentist.

Next, decide whether you would like to quit right after selling or allow yourself the right to continue practicing dentistry in your practice for as long as you'd like after the sale, but without the hassle of ownership. Under these conditions you could take a month off for that long-awaited vacation. You could practice dentistry for two or three days a week and still make a lot of money, and you could have a week off every other week if you'd like to have it. Also, you could practice for three or four hours a day if you wish. Just about everything and anything is possible when your practice no longer owns you. You are free at last!

There are some of you that would like to sell and get your total practice value out now (while prices are high and taxes are low) and continue in an ownership position after the sale. That's right...you can be paid for the entire value of your practice now and still carry on as an equal owner of your practice after the sale, for as many years as you'd like! You would share the responsibilities of managing the practice, you could cut back on the number of workdays, take a lot more time off and still be paid for providing dental services, plus 50% of the profits generated by your practice for as long as you'd like. Imagine being paid for the full value of your practice and continuing to be paid 50% of the profits generated by your practice for years to come!

So, it's up to you to sell your practice now and lock in the value of your practice to secure your financial future.

The Big Question: How Much Money Do I Need?

Your future spending will likely be similar to your current spending. Knowing this, you can calculate how much money you'll need to retire. Here's the best shot I've heard to helping you figure this out-- you will need somewhere between **20 to 30 times** your annual spending. The older you are, the lower you can go on this spectrum. The younger you are, the higher you'll need to go on the spectrum. That's easy enough, right?

Just take what you spend annually and multiply it by 30:

Current Income $_____

times 20 - 30 equals

$_____ **Retirement Needed**

This figure will represent how much money you need for a successful retirement. Everything you have accumulated excluding your home. We don't count your home because you must have a place to live and most people don't want to have debt on their home when they retire. To determine how much you have accumulated, use the following calculations.

Cash $_____
Investments $_____
Real estate equity $_____
Practice equity $_____
_____ $_____
_____ $_____
_____ $_____
TOTAL Retirement $_____

Subtract Retirement Needed $_____

If **TOTAL Retirement** is more than **Retirement Needed**, then you are ready to retire. If it is less than **Retirement Needed**, then begin now to grow your available funds to generate the retirement you have dreamed about all those years you have been working while anticipating those "Golden Years".

Just imagine: You can extract the $500,000 - $1,000,000 in equity value out of your practice and have all the benefits you enjoy in your practice while giving all the things you do not enjoy to a younger colleague who would take care of the rest of the responsibilities of your practice.

Case Study
Dr. A in Arizona had accumulated enough assets to be able to retire per his Financial Planner. He still enjoyed the clinical part of dentistry, so he decided to sell his practice on a pre-sale so that he could continue to do the clinical dentistry he wanted to do. He began to accept only the cosmetic cases, which were his favorite, while referring the other procedures

to the purchaser of his practice. The purchaser was excited to receive those referrals as it was a great opportunity to get to know the new patients. Dr. sold his practice for $700,000, which only made his retirement sweeter. He continued to practice but, only 2 ½ days per week. His paychecks after the sale were $12,000 to $20,000 depending upon whether he took extended vacations or not. He chose to work a schedule that provided him with a 6-day vacation twice a month as well.

As you can see, retirement takes on a whole new meaning when you see it from a new perspective. If you are financially secure, then you have some great options available to you. If you think you don't have enough money set aside to retire and would like to get out of the hassle of ownership, there are programs that can help you too.

After 50 years of working with dentists, we alone have developed over *150 programs* that are needed to provide you with options that best fit your needs at this critical time of your life. Contact the authors to begin your road to 'Finishing Rich' at 480-634-4803 or www.aftco.net.

Chapter 3

What Type of Transition Should I Use?

If you fail to plan, you are planning to fail!
Benjamin Franklin

Planning...everyone keeps talking to you about planning for your future and you've barely enough time to take care of present issues. Who has time to plan? Retirement? That's light years from now. Besides that, who is going to retire? You plan to work if your health holds out, so you don't need to plan for retirement.

Why worry? You are as healthy as a horse. Disability? Well, you've got that well covered with disability insurance. Sure, you'd have to make some adjustments in your lifestyle if you became disabled, but who wouldn't? (Maybe you'd better find those old disability policies and read them over again.)

The quality of life is more important than life itself.
Alexis Carrel

Quality of Life Scheduling

What is it? Well, it is different for every dentist, but for some it can be described as "doing dentistry because you want to, doing only those procedures you enjoy, and doing them only on those patients you wish to treat and only when you want to be working"!

This also can be interpreted as "freedom." Most doctors would prefer to spend less time in the office (rather than more time), so it's safe to say that taking more time off and having the financial resources to spend more time traveling, hunting, fishing, golf, etc., will improve your Quality of Life! Have you ever been with someone who was on their deathbed who said, "I wish I had spent more time at the office?"

Overhead, however, is a 365-day fact of life for every practice owner and takes up between 50% to 60% of annual gross revenues. Doctors cannot practice every day of the year, so they practice five days a week which allows them to generate enough income to pay the overhead expenses and to pay themselves reasonable compensation as well.

So, when a doctor decides to back down to a 4-day work week, they don't think about how this affects their net income. A 4-day work week or, for that matter, a 3-day work week is fantastic, but the problem is the practice still has the same 365 days overhead. You can cut your hours back, but you cannot cut staff salaries or rent, utilities, telephone and all the other fixed expenses of the practice.

If you practice 5 days a week and have a 60% overhead, then the first 3 days of income pays the overhead expenses. The remaining 2 days of practice income represents the doctor's compensation and profit. When you cut to a 4-day work week, there is less time to produce revenue for the practice, and the overhead expenses remain the same.

Cutting to a 4-day work week means you now only have one day of production to pay the doctor's compensation (remember, it takes 3 days to pay the overhead). When you drop one day from your work schedule, you lower your time in the office by 20%, but you will also find that you have a 50% drop in personal income for the doctor. Obviously, cutting back to a 4-day work week is great from a Quality of Life standpoint, but it could be a financial disaster.

We have developed a "Quality of Life Scheduling Program" for doctors who no longer want to practice 5 days a week. However, instead of going to a 4-day week, which is a mistake, the doctor should consider a 3-day schedule which provides a better Quality of Life because you now have more time off to enjoy all the things you've always wanted to experience, without a drop-in income.

This program is designed to keep the practice open 5 days a week. The owner practices only 3 days a week, but the office is open 5 days a week. This is done by adding another doctor to the practice! That's right, one practice with two doctors, each scheduling 3 work days per week with an overlapping day. Both doctors practice a 3 day a week schedule, but the office is open for the entire 5 days. This controls office overhead and it increases overall practice profitability.

Another nice feature is that you are available to your patients all 5 days (Monday thru Friday), it's just a matter of which week you will be available for that day of the week. Also, you will enjoy a 6-day vacation every other week while in this program! This will considerably improve the Quality of Life for both doctors and control overhead at the same time.

Believe it or not, most doctors could see and treat all their patients in just 3 days a week. The only reason the office is open 4 or 5 days a week is most doctors cannot stand the idea of paying the full-time staff salaries... and have them work less than full time. Thus, the staff schedule the patients over that 4 or 5 days to justify their salaries, and the doctor subjects himself/herself to a 4 or 5-day work schedule! Well, with our Quality of Life Scheduling program, the staff will work their full 5 days each week, so you can go to sleep each night knowing they are not getting one up on you.

If you have more patients than you can see in 3 days, then you probably have more patients than you need to be seeing by yourself. That's right; you should be able to produce more than enough income on the number of patients you can see in just three days a week. If you have an excess of patients, then you have even more scheduling options as to how this program can be implemented in your practice. This could include a practice merger, an associate/partnership program, a sale, purchase, or a combination of any one of these options.

Pre-Sale Program

The Pre-Sale Program was developed for the dentist who has built a successful practice over the years and now wants to realize its maximum financial benefits, while preparing for retirement and/or a career change sometime in the future.

Through the implementation of the Pre-Sale Program, the seller can continue to work in the practice for a pre-determined number of years and enjoy the following benefits:

PERSONAL FREEDOM: You sell your practice and have the right to continue to work in the practice for as many years as you wish (pre-determined by you). You are then free of those costly overhead expenses that prevented you from having the time to pursue other interests or enjoying those well-deserved vacations.

CONTINUOUS INCOME: As the years go by and you'd like to slow down, you can always enjoy a "positive cash flow" because you are no longer responsible for practice overhead. Your income is assured regardless of how little you practice since you are paid a fixed percentage of your collected production, no matter how much or how little that may be.

PRACTICE VALUE PROTECTION: Your practice is sold while at its peak value so that asset is protected from a declining practice value that would result from your untimely death or disability. Selling at peak value eliminates the need for your family to attempt to sell your practice at a time of great personal loss.

INTEREST INCOME: Your passive income will be substantially increased by converting a non-interest bearing asset (your practice) into an interest-bearing asset after the sale (return on investment from the proceeds of the sale of your practice).

CONFIDENTIALITY: The transaction remains confidential until you are ready to retire. At the time of the sale, we merely announce the transaction as either an association or a practice merger, not a sale.

TRANSITION: Introducing another professional to your patients, years before your eventual retirement, allows for a smooth transition as you phase out of practice. Your patients can become familiar with your new colleague, reassuring them of continuous care once you elect to retire. Once you have completed this transaction, you will gain an entirely new and refreshing perspective on your profession. You will have the option of practicing when you want, on who you want, and be doing only the procedures you want to do.

Pension Funding

You've done better than most. Your friends and colleagues hold you in high regard. Your family is appreciative of how you have provided for them over the years. You don't have a bad track record and you have reason to be proud. However, there may be one very important item that was compromised in your quest to provide so much for so many-- your pension plan.

You figured out how to get into practice and be a success. Now, at your age, it's time to figure out how you can get out of practice...alive. You don't want to practice until you die because you cannot afford to retire. You don't want death to be your reward for a lifetime of providing for others. You want a chance to enjoy life now. We are talking about freedom from stress and quality of life.

It takes a great deal of money to do this. However, chances

are that you are working as hard as you want at this stage in your life, and you are probably spending almost all your earnings just to maintain your present lifestyle. Putting money away for retirement is a great idea provided it does not require you to work longer hours or lower your current standard of living.

You may still have to incur some future college expenses for your children, and the house may still have a substantial mortgage payment. You figure that you need to practice for at least another ten years or so just to make ends meet and that puts you even closer to retirement age, so where can you get the money you need for your pension plan?

Your practice! It is one asset that can be liquidated now and the value of your practice utilized to fund your pension plan. You can cash in on the value of your practice now and continue to practice for five, ten or even fifteen years (you determine the number of years, of course). This unique program will allow you to contribute that money to your pension plan for your benefit only (no staff contributions).

What happens next is interesting. Once we complete this program for you and the money begins to flow the miracle of compound interest takes over. Interest is paid on principal and interest is paid on interest, and that money in your pension plan begins to grow at a rapid rate. By the time you are ready to retire, the money you received for the value of your practice could grow by two, three and even four times the present value of your practice. That compounded value should more than adequately provide for your retirement and you did not have to compromise your lifestyle.

Now, suppose you decide to do nothing and continue as you have been. You will work another ten years or so (provided you don't die or become disabled in the interim), and you probably still won't have the money set aside for retirement. So, you might try to lower your standard of living to save money. You may begin by selling your house and moving into a smaller one. The problem is, it will also be more difficult at that age to maintain today's level of production. Thus, your income may begin to drop as well. There goes the extra money for retirement, even after you lower your standard of living.

The only option left is to work until you die. If you die, you have life insurance to take care of your estate. If you get sick and can't work, however, that is a whole different picture (and not a very pretty one). You would not believe the number of doctors we've seen retire over the years that did so just hoping they would die before their money ran out!

This does not have to happen to you, however, because you can do something about it.

Using any of the 150 transition plans we've created, you can have your cake and eat it too! Imagine continuing to practice as long as you desire and having your retirement funds doubling every 10 years. Remove the stress of your practice and retain only the parts you truly enjoy. You can continue your present income, fund your retirement plan and improve your quality of life NOW. Don't put it off, call us today 480-634-4803 or visit www.aftco.net to arrange for a FREE consultation. You will be glad you did!

Chapter 4

How to Determine Practice Value

"Price is what you pay, value is what you get"
Warren Buffet

Practice values are at an all-time high right now! What does this mean for your dental practice though? How can you capture the greatest value for your practice? A lot of doomsayers want you to believe practice values are currently low with all the options in dentistry today. They'll say practices sell for 65% of one year's collections or they might say things like the practice is too old to be sold. We've sold offices for over 100% of collections in some cases and had to choose which buyer got the practice! The reality is that for most doctors graduating today their only option for a sustainable financial future is practice ownership. This has greatly increased the value of dental practices in high demand areas. The value in your practice comes from finding the RIGHT purchaser and then presenting the opportunity in a way that highlights the value you have created.

The more turn key the opportunity the greater value it has. If you find the RIGHT purchaser and transition it correctly, you WILL get the highest value for your practice! In this chapter, you will learn what contributes to the value of a dental practice as well as how to create a quick valuation on your practice.

Case Study:

After practicing for over 30 years Dr. Bill decided it was time to make a change. The problem was his practice had been declining about 10% every year for the last 5 years. He kept thinking, "if I can grow my practice I'll be able to get more value out of it". His financials for retirement weren't very strong so he was relying on the sale of his practice for retirement. Unfortunately, he thought, "I can work a few more years and make more money than selling now." He continued to work for another 3 years and each year continued to decline in revenue. The practice had declined so much that his profits were deep in the red. This meant he had to cut his own salary significantly every year just to keep the lights on. If Bill had sold when his revenue had peaked, worked for the buyer as an associate and put the proceeds from the sale into a pension plan option he could have created a retirement worth enjoying. Bill was so distraught about selling to a new doctor that he let go of his retirement and was left with a practice that had little to no value and very little assets and options for retirement. This all stemmed from the emotional decision of not selling his practice and not knowing what would happen to his patients and staff. Rest assured that if you find the RIGHT purchaser they will treat your patients and staff with the best care possible as they don't want to jeopardize their future success in the practice. There are hundreds of ways to transition a practice based on your financial needs now and in the future. There is no need to delay this process especially if your story is like Bill's. Get started on planning for your future because if you fail to plan, plan to fail.

Practice value is defined as the amount a willing seller and willing buyer come to an agreement on. This can be a positive or a negative depending on the intentions of both parties. If the parties are focused on getting the highest or lowest price neither one of them will get the highest value for the practice. As Warren Buffet states, "Price is what you pay, value is what you get." The price of a dental practice is only a very small part of determining the actual value of a dental practice. So how do you determine the "value" of your dental practice? There are a lot of contributing factors that determine value and we will get into these later in this chapter. For now, let's start with the basics and discuss where the true "value" in a dental practice is and how you can maximize this for the buyer...thus increasing your price.

First, we need to identify what creates value in your dental practice. In every practice, there are intangible and tangible assets. The greatest value in any practice is the goodwill between you and your patients and you and your staff. These are the intangible assets that will hold the greatest value. The tangible assets will include things like equipment, supplies, etc... The main contributing factors that determine practice value are: Profitability, Patient base, Staff, Demographics (both internally and externally), and Equipment. These five factors will give you the greatest impact when determining the value of your practice. These can increase or decrease your practice valuation.

1) Let's start with the profitability as it is the most critical when determining the viability of your practice. To determine this, you will need to have a copy of the last full year's P&L or Tax Return for the practice. If your CPA has done a good job minimizing your taxes, then you are likely not showing much profit to minimize taxes. A purchaser will want to review your business tax returns to determine what they will

expect to make after the purchase. Now think about explaining this unprofitability to a buyer-candidate if your financials haven't been prepared for a future sale.

The first step is to categorize real and elective expenses from the information on your tax returns that explain the "true, profitability" of your practice. Elective expenses are classified as expenses not needed to run the actual practice. Examples are: auto, life insurance, excessive C.E., travel, etc. A properly ran practice in the metro area should have a 56%-60% overhead without paying the dentist. In a rural area (less than 500,000 people) the overhead should be closer to 50%-55% without paying the dentist. If your overhead is higher, then that will decrease the price of your practice. If the overhead is lower, it is an increasing factor for your sales price.

2) The second factor is determining your patient base. This includes your active patient base and new patient flow each month. An active patient is defined as any patient that has received treatment from your practice within the last 24 months (36 in a rural area). This includes emergency patients as well. If you have paper charts you can hand count each one or an easier and faster way that will get you a fairly accurate count is to count one row of charts and then multiple by the number of rows you have. An example would be if you have 100 charts in a row and you have 10 rows of charts you can conclude that you have around 1,000 active patients in your practice. This is all dependent though on each chart being marked correctly. If you are all digital, then first pat yourself on the back for keeping up with current technology then call your support line to get directions on how to pull up the active patient count. Each practice

software and version is different so the quickest way for you to do this is to get them on the phone and walk you through how to get the report. Typically, this only takes a couple minutes and will significantly show the value of your practice opportunity.

Analyzing the potential in your practice is another factor to have ready for a potential candidate. This shows the buyer what the potential future growth is in an office. This is done by determining the annual production per patient and then comparing it to the industry averages or comparing it to the buyer's production per patient. Production per patient is calculated by taking the Net Collections of the practice and dividing that by the number of active patients in the practice. An active patient is defined as any patient seen in the last 24 months at least one or more times. Below is the formula so you can enter your data to give you a baseline for your practice.

Production Per Patient Formula:

_____ / _____ = _____

Practice Collections *(divided by)* Active Patients Prod. per Patient per Year

New patient flow is critical for the future sustainability of the practice. Your new patient flow is what regulates or increases the attrition every dental practice has on an annual basis. The average practice across the country has an attrition of 20% per year. This means if you have 1,000 active patients, 200 patients will not be returning. To maintain your patient base, you will need to bring in another 200 active patients from either internal or external marketing sources. If you can't mitigate this attrition, then you will expect to see an annual drop each year in your revenue which in turn will decrease the value of your practice. This is an area that I see a lot of offices losing practice value. This is getting to be an increasingly difficult problem for many private practice owners as there are a lot of competition out there with corporate groups, private equity firms, multiple practice owners and even Wal-Mart is talking about opening dental practices in many of their locations. Private practice owners don't have the resources to compete with corporate giants and in turn have had to go to more creative ways to market to new patients.

3) Staff is another critical factor that will determine the value in a dental practice. Having a trained staff that has created years of goodwill with your patients will only enhance the value of your practice. Buyers are willing to pay more for an office with a good core team in place that has a strong relationship with the patients and all work together with little to no drama. I've seen offices drop in value within minutes when staff turnover happens. There is another side to this as well though. Staff costs should hover between 22%-26% of total revenue. If your team has been getting raises each year and the revenue has stagnated for the last 10-20 years, then the staff costs will quickly get out of line. In some cases, we have seen staff salaries be as high as 40% of revenue. There are two ways to fix this issue:

A. You can reduce salaries and reduce benefits, or if you're over staffed, then you can eliminate positions that are no longer needed for the size of your practice. I don't get many doctors wanting to do this so they are more in favor for the second option.

B. Increase revenue of your practice. This is easier said than done but if you can increase the revenue of your practice then the staff salaries will fall in line where they should be.

4) The 4th determining factor is the demographics inside and outside your practice. The highest value practices are ones where the internal demographics are comparable to the demographics of patients around the practice. If a doctor owns a high fee cosmetic office in low income area, then the potential growth of that practice is limited to what is being seen in the practice already. The risk to a buyer is that they will not be able to maintain the revenue of the practice in a declining neighborhood. This risk then reduces the price of the practice as it's not a maintainable practice. The key to this section is to ensure the practice you own matches the demographics around. If your practice has been declining the last few years quickly look at the demographics around your practice and determine if your practice is outside the market conditions now.

5) The final main factor to consider is the equipment in an office. A lot of reps will lead you to believe that buying brand new equipment right before retirement is the right thing to do. Unfortunately, this advice typically costs doctors tens and even hundreds of thousands of dollars. Yes, having newer equipment might incentivize a buyer to look at the practice but the dollars you spend on new equipment will never be realized in the sale.
It's a general rule of thumb that new dental equipment is worth less than 25% to a valuation when it is installed. If you spend $50,000 in new equipment it will likely only add about

$10,000 - $20,000 in additional value. The exception to this is more expensive equipment like a Cerec or Cone Beam CT Scanner. It is like painting your house before a sale. It might help it sell faster but it won't increase the value much if any at all. Your practice price will be higher but after paying the debt on the new equipment you will be negative equity in it. A general rule is to keep all your equipment running and in working order so the new buyer will be able to at least maintain the practice. If the practice has good cash flow a buyer can always buy new equipment later. Plus, most buyers will want their own specific equipment and what you purchase might not be what they're looking for.

Now with all of this taken into consideration we can run an initial Valuation of your practice. Below is a quick valuation tool for you to get a general idea of your practice price. There are other factors that determine the full practice value so take that into consideration as it might increase or decrease the full value of your office depending on your circumstances. Every practice is unique and requires a full valuation to determine the exact value in today's dental market.

The type of transition strategy you use to sell your practice will also determine the practice value. If it is a high-risk transition for the buyer, then the value would be lower than if it's a lower risk transition. Positioning your practice with the right strategy for you and the buyer is instrumental in getting the highest value for your practice.

The example below is a Fee for Service practice in a metro area with new equipment and a good location. This office also has a low overhead with good staff management. As you can see this office is collecting $1,700,000 and has a valuation of 92%. This would price the practice around $1,564,000 for a normal transition.

Demographics	Rural Metro	18.0% 30.0%	30.0%
Practice Type	Medicaid G.P. FFS/PPO G.P.	5.0% 18.0%	18.0%
Equipment/ office decor	>10 years old <10 years old	7.0% 12.0%	12.0%
Office Location	Bad Good	5.0% 10.0%	10.0%
Overhead	>60% <60%	10.0% 20.0%	20.0%
Staff	>25% <25%	-2.0% 2.0%	2.0%
Value		TOTAL	92%
Annual Practice Collections (last 12 months)	$1,700,000	Multiply the percentage in "TOTAL" above to give you the practice value	$1,564,000

Here is a blank form so you can input your practice data to complete an initial valuation on your practice:

Demographics	Rural Metro	18.0% 30.0%	
Practice Type	Medicaid G.P. FFS/PPO G.P.	5.0% 18.0%	
Equipment/ office decor	>10 years old <10 years old	7.0% 12.0%	
Office Location	Bad Good	5.0% 10.0%	
Overhead	>60% <60%	10.0% 20.0%	
Staff	>25% <25%	-2.0% 2.0%	
Value		TOTAL	
Annual Practice Collections (last 12 months)		Multiply the percentage in "TOTAL" above to give you the practice value	

Now that you have a ballpark figure of your practice price, the next step is to create a strategy to get a buyer to be willing to pay it. Educating the buyer is critical in getting full value for your practice. Here at AFTCO we spend countless hours with the buyer before a transition occurs to teach them what to look for in an office as well as helping them understand the value you've created in your practice.

Keep in mind the other categories that will determine the valuation as well, and only someone in touch with the market will be able to complete. Things like supply & demand, current market trends, transition options, seller financing options, etc. This valuation tool is meant to be used to give you an initial idea of the value of your practice. To get a FREE full practice valuation visit www.aftco.net or call 480-634-4803 today!

Chapter 5

The Transition Process

"Coming together is a beginning; keeping together is progress; working together is success."
Henry Ford

So far, we've covered the foundation of determining where you are in the process, your personal needs & goals, as well as how to quickly complete a valuation on your practice. Next up is understanding the purchaser and process of a transition.

So, what is a buyer looking for in a practice? What is the buyer expecting from me throughout the transition process? How will the buyer see the value in my practice? How will I know when I have found the right buyer? What do I do if things become adversarial? How do I complete a transition? Believe me, we've heard these questions and many other concerns from EVERY seller we work with. If you're thinking this way, then you are going to be asking the right questions throughout the process.

Case Study:
Dr. Fred graduated dental school in 2012. Right out of school he found an associate position for an office in Mesa, AZ and was very excited to begin working. After all he had just completed almost 10 years of post-high school education and was ready to enter his chosen profession. Soon after starting he realized there just wasn't enough

dentistry to do to keep him busy. He was averaging $130,000 per year in personal income but he was barely getting by with the mountain of school debt and other debt that allowed him to get through school. He quickly realized he needed to find something better. After some serious searching, he realized that even the average associate in the country makes $148,000 per year. He was at a very serious turning point in his career. Does he just accept what is normal in dentistry and try to make it work or does he go out and find something better? That's when I got the call to meet with him. After an in-depth analysis of his finances, needs and goals we decided practice ownership was the best way for him to get out of the hole he had dug (like many dentists graduating today). I located an office in Phoenix, AZ that after paying the bills and paying the seller he would net over $250,000! The office sold for 92% of collections and Fred was more than happy to pay it. After all, his income would almost double as the owner. The added benefit is with his enthusiasm and energy in growing the practice he now takes home over $500,000 per year.

So, why am I telling you a story about a young buyer out of school? The main reason is to show you that the office sold for 92% because there was a willing buyer and the practice was the future stability for the doctor's family. He didn't think about the price even once when he realized the current income and future potential of the practice. He saw this as HIS future practice and not just another practice for sale. If a buyer doesn't see the value in what they are purchasing, then the price will be the only factor they are focused on. Find the *RIGHT* buyer and with the right transition plan, it will truly be a win-win scenario. Having someone who knows how to navigate the transition and ensure you get the highest value for your practice is priority #1.

This chapter is to serve as an understanding of the current mental and financial state of most first-time purchasers as well as the brief overview of the transition process. Other purchasers, though, include corporate groups, private equity firms, venture capitalists, non-dentists (in some states) and dentists owning multiple practices. Since first time purchasers represent the highest percentage of purchasers, we will focus on them.

Most first-time purchasers have these 9 characteristics:
1. Graduated from dental school 1-7 years ago
2. Have over $400,000 in student debt
3. Tired of working for someone else
4. Want to be their own boss
5. Want a better quality of life
6. Want long term financial stability for their family
7. Want to practice within 30 minutes of their home
8. Typically have no assets or means to pay for the practice without bank funding
9. Not making enough money in their current position

Having seen this now, you can quickly realize the position of most dentists that are working for someone else. Understanding the purchaser is pivotal in understanding how to show the value of your practice opportunity. If your practice opportunity meets these criteria for the purchaser, then it will likely equal a successful transition.

This is a flowchart of the average practice transition:

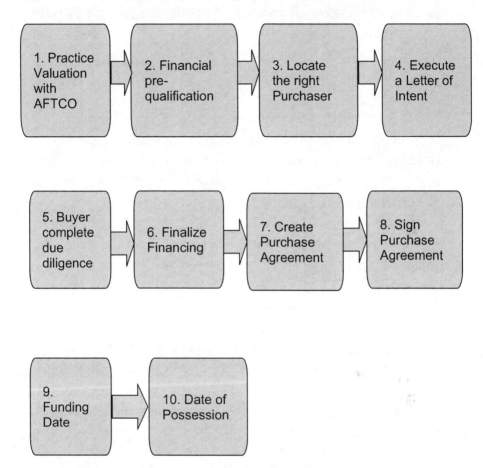

What is the General Transition Process?

This is the general process from start to finish. Did you know that less than 10% of doctor to doctor transitions are ever completed? Even typical practice brokers that use adversarial negotiations and one sided transitions only close around 22% and at a much lower price than originally presented. Whereas our company holds a closing rate of well over 92%.

This is done through our unique transition process and vetting candidates to ensure that they are a good match for you and your practice.

Locate the Right Purchaser

There are many ways to locate a purchaser. Modern technology allows you to connect with a tremendous number of people in a very quick time. If you're not the type to sit down and publish ads for your practice, then there are other options as well. To get full value for your practice, the right buyer will be one that is well educated on the transition process as well as one that understands the true value of your practice. This can be the difference between a smooth transition where you get top dollar for your office or an adversarial transition where the buyer negotiates throughout the entire process and nickels and dimes you on everything. I've seen sellers face both buyer types and the sellers that deal with the negotiated buyers almost always end up losing thousands and thousands of dollars due to not understanding the process and just allowing the buyer to have what they want.

Financial Pre-Qualification

Before spending too much time with a candidate for your practice it is important to know their ability to get funding on your practice. It's much better to find this out at the beginning rather than at the end once you've invested time and money with this purchaser. There are hundreds of lenders funding dental practice loans and it is critical the right one is chosen or you might be looking at significant carryback on your practice. As an example, we once had a bank only willing to fund 50% of the loan. We took that same practice, transition, buyer & seller to a separate bank and could get **FULL** financing for the buyer. Which in turn meant the seller was given 100% of his purchase price at time of funding.

Complete Due Diligence

Due diligence is the time that allows the buyer to investigate and review the practice financials, reports, schedule, charts and much more. It is critical that the buyer know what they are looking at or they will likely end up getting paralysis by analysis and will never decide on purchasing. Or worse, they will say "no" just out of misunderstanding and fear. This is also the time that you can review info on the buyer to ensure he is the right candidate for your practice.

Finalize Financing

The bank will require many items from you, your CPA and from your practice to determine the viability of the practice for the buyer. We typically go to a minimum of three banks to get funding done in today's world. The 2008 recession hurt a lot of people and dentistry wasn't exempt from it. This left many banks needing bailouts from bad loans. Since then, the banks have had to tighten up their lending parameters and are very specific to the types of transitions they want to do. Knowing which bank to use is critical in today's financial climate.

Sign Contracts

Once the price, terms, banking and due diligence has been

completed, then the next step is to get a drafted contract. It is critical to have someone with dental transition experience handling this as we've seen tens of thousands of dollars lost as well as terrible terms agreed to just for the sake of completing a transition. In one case, we had a seller spend over $20,000 on an attorney to draft a contract that the buyer never agreed to which resulted in a failed transition. The buyer went on to acquire another office and the seller to this day has never sold his practice due to unreasonable terms for a buyer.

Funding Date

The funding date is defined as the date that money changes hands between the buyer and seller. Typically, there is 1-2 weeks between the funding date and the buyer taking possession. This allows time for the buyer to meet the staff and tie up any other loose ends that couldn't be completed until after funding.

Take Possession

Congratulations! This is the time when the purchaser takes over physical possession of the practice. From here on out the purchaser will handle the management and day to day operations of the practice.

Other Considerations While Working with A Buyer

1. Confidentiality is #1 when you are considering selling your practice. As a rule, the fewer people that know about the sale the better. This goes for your staff as well. As we discussed earlier the staff is a key determination of the value of your practice. We've seen staff that finds out about the sale begin looking for new jobs immediately after as they assume the buyer will fire them when they take over. This is rarely the case as an educated buyer will understand the value your staff has in the practice and will rely on their expertise in growing the practice.

2. Honesty is the best policy. Your mother said it when you were young and I'm saying it again. This should go without saying but the key to a successful transition is both sides being open and honest about the practice and their intentions. Most of the time when a seller tries to hide something the buyer figures it out in due diligence (If they're a competent buyer). And if they don't figure it out then you likely wouldn't want them working with your staff or patients anyways.

3. Know your practice or hire someone that will present it correctly. Perception is everything in the initial stages of a transition. If the perception is negative, then a great opportunity might go for pennies on the dollar. If the perception is positive, then you will be fighting off candidates for your practice as they will be coming in droves.

4. There is a right buyer for every practice! If the buyer you have currently interested isn't giving you the "warm fuzzies" then move on to a better candidate. There are so many doctors looking for practices that there is no need to try and fit a square peg in a round hole. If you try to sell the practice to the wrong purchaser, then the purchase price becomes the primary focus rather than the uniqueness of the practice opportunity. This leads to prolonged negotiations, wounded pride, hurt feelings, and both parties feeling that their needs were compromised; and this is a lousy way to sell a practice.

5. Every practice is unique and needs a different transition plan for the seller. If the purchaser doesn't meet your transition plan, then you have the wrong purchaser. Again, don't force it. If it's meant to be it will and if it's not, then it won't.

6. If you live in a high demand area, then it is likely a seller's market. Don't let anyone tell you any differently unless they have experience in transitioning practices. Even then there should be specific reasons as to why it's not. Reasons like estate sales, disability, malpractice, etc.

7. Don't sacrifice your future for the sake of completing a transition. There are good practices and there are some that are not so good. Practices with low revenues, no profits, few patients are better off being sold and merged with another office near you. If the right strategy for the practice is taken, then the value will increase.

Imagine for a second what type of buyer you are looking for. Does your practice meet the criteria we discussed for the buyer? If it does, then you have now created the initial footprint of the type of candidate that will fit your practice. Keep in mind that there is no perfect purchaser just like there is no perfect practice. The key is to determine the type of person you are looking for and then with the help of an expert determining if the candidate can learn the aspects of dentistry they might not know yet. Specifically, management.

Most buyers have little to no business experience and aren't equipped to manage the office right out of school. Even after a long-term associate position they are given little experience in running a practice. Unfortunately, the best teacher is experience. We can coach them along the way as well as get them in touch with other people that can assist them while they navigate through ownership. Even with the doctor's limited experience, we're told the default rate with most banks is under 1%. That's a pretty safe investment if you ask us.

At AFTCO, we have helped dentists achieve successful transitions for over 50 years across the country. We do this by educating the buyer candidates to fully understand the true value of what you have created in your practice. This tried and proven system has worked for thousands of dentists and well over $3.2 Billion in practice sales. To learn more about our transition system, call 480-634-4803 or visit www.aftco.net.

Chapter 6

Do's and Don'ts of Selling Your Practice

*"Give me six hours to chop down a tree and
I will spend the first four sharpening the axe."*
Abraham Lincoln

Now that you've considered your options along with figuring out which option intrigue you the most, we now need to discuss basic etiquette when preparing your practice for a future sale. What if I told you that good preparation could increase your practice value by as much as 10%-20%? Like selling a home or car, there are many things you should do and many things you shouldn't do. So, how do you determine what should and should not be done? What factors increase or decrease the value of a dental office or the perceived value from the buyer? What is a buyer looking for on the first visit and every visit thereafter? How will you know when your practice is "presentation" ready? These are all questions we intend to answer for you in this chapter!

Let's think about buying a used car, as just about everyone has bought a used car at some point in their life. We have a friend that owns a car dealership and he explained all the steps it takes to get a car "sales ready". We were blown away at how much is done to make a small profit on a car. They have over 20 processes and a handful of employees that get this car ready before even considering putting it back on the lot for sale. Now apply this to your dental practice-- how much prep are you willing to do to make the practice look and feel like it is worth the millions of dollars?

It's the age-old struggle of getting the buyer to see the intangible value in your office that you've come to love. In most cases your staff and patients have been with you since you can remember and are valued as high as family. How do you sell a relationship to an interested candidate? The key is in the presentation to the buyer along with the perception the doctor sees and feels when he walks into the office. The other key that a lot of people don't talk about is your ability to sell your staff's skills and worth to the buyer candidate. If done correctly the buyer will rely on the staff in helping him get transitioned into the practice. If done poorly the buyer could see little value in the staff and will be looking to replace them if they aren't doing things "his" way.

There are hundreds if not thousands of Do's & Don'ts for your practice so we are going to touch on the major ones that we see on a regular basis. To come up with the list, we have reviewed countless transitions, as well as information from doctors that have tried to do it on their own as well.

The following categories we will be reviewing are the most common mistakes that most dentists make when transitioning the practice themselves or with an inexperienced broker. We will have 6 categories: Staff, Facility, Equipment, Marketing, Revenue & Profit and Meeting the Buyer.

Staff

DO: Confidentiality is vital in a transition as the transition risk rises if staff and patients find out about the sale. You can assume that anytime the transition risk rises the practice value decreases. We don't want the staff to seek employment elsewhere because they may think the buyer will replace them or worse that you will just pick up and leave the practice without a replacement. It is preferable to wait and tell your staff about the sale once the sale is final. It is ideal to tell the staff with the new buyer being present so they can answer questions from the staff as well as put their minds at ease about their jobs. This can be a very emotional time for staff so be ready to see some water works and general sadness about the change.

However, if the staff or one of your trusted staff members suspect something, then have a meeting with them (or preferably just that one staff person) and tell them your plans (retirement, career move, etc.). Inform them that you have retained someone to locate a purchaser for the practice. You can assure them that you are making every effort to find another doctor for the practice and that their jobs are secure. Be very positive when discussing the sale with the staff, letting them know that you are looking out for their future by seeing to it that the practice will continue after your retirement! Expect them to be somewhat sad and concerned about whom the purchaser will be, but you should assure them that you will do your best to see that a suitable replacement is located.

NOTE: In most cases the staff and their salaries generally are secure following the sale unless certain staff members are uncooperative (which usually does not happen because they want to keep their jobs).

DO NOT: tell the staff that the practice is for sale until we have located a purchaser and closed the transaction, if possible. Do not promise them a job with the purchaser, even though you can feel confident that their job is secure. Do not increase salaries or benefits just before a closing without notifying the purchaser.

Facility

DO: Straighten up and clean your office. The waiting room makes the first impression, so see to it that your staff makes an extra effort to clean it before leaving at night. The magazines in the waiting room should be current. If you have a lab, then see that the equipment and counters are clean and uncluttered. There is no need for making leasehold improvements such as painting and replacing the carpet.

If you own the building, then be certain that the area around the building is neatly mowed and bushes trimmed and make any necessary repairs to the parking lot.

DO NOT: Buy new equipment or make any expensive leasehold improvements. Please do not promise the potential purchaser that you will be replacing or making leasehold improvements; the purchaser will be prepared for what he or she will see in your office. We base the sale on the economic value of the transaction, not the value of the tangible assets. Too much emphasis on the equipment etc. works against completing a successful transaction.

Equipment

Do Not: Many people would like you to believe that buying brand new fancy equipment will quickly increase the value of your practice. Unfortunately, there are very few exceptions where this is true. For example, at the time of this writing a slightly used Cerec can be purchased on eBay for around $30,000. Brand new these retail for around $150,000. Dental equipment in general depreciates faster than any other asset you might own even your car.

Do: The exception to buying equipment is when your existing equipment is so outdated and run down that a buyer couldn't practice dentistry there even if they tried. In this case begin looking at used equipment or refurbished equipment that you can cheaply outfit your practice with more current technology. Before any purchases are made ($2,500+) I recommend consulting with an expert to see what the value will be when you decide to sell your office.

Marketing

Do Not: Don't decrease your marketing budget right before a sale. Nothing is more demotivating to a buyer than seeing the new patient flow take a big dive right before they take over the practice. Remember, the idea when transitioning your practice is to make it as turnkey as possible for the new buyer. The better the opportunity for the buyer the higher value you can receive for your practice.

Do: It is best to compile material used for your marketing plans to showcase it to potential buyers. This allows you to show them what has and hasn't worked in your attempts to bring in new patients. If the buyer can see a clear way to continue to grow the practice the more confident they will be in moving forward. Buyer confidence is instrumental in achieving a successful win-win transition. The more confident the buyer the better he/she will feel about your practice.

Revenue & Profit

Do Not: Let the revenue or profits decline the last 3-5 years of ownership. I had a doctor once in a small town decide to sell his office. We determined that based on his location it would likely take 1-2 years to sell his office. The doctor decided to let "senioritis" kick in and just relax the last year of ownership. He had a strong practice collecting around $1,400,000 and within 12 months the revenue dropped to $900,000. This cost the doctor almost $400,000 in equity due to the decline. Now you may be thinking, "that could never happen to my practice" but unfortunately, we see it happen often. Typically, the last 5-10 years of ownership are the least productive for most offices. This in turn increases the overhead which resulting in lower profitability for the office. As mentioned earlier profitability is a key component when evaluating a dental office. If the profitability shrinks, then the value shrinks.

Do: The moral of that story is to make sure that you have a strategy over the next 5-10 years to ensure your revenue continues to rise. The practice that have gotten the highest values have been the ones that we have worked with to safeguard the revenue and profitability. If you're feeling tired, bored or aren't as excited about dentistry as you were when you graduated dental school then those are the first signs of a future decline in revenue.

Meeting the Buyer

DO: discuss your practice philosophy and methods of treatment. Disclose any unique or unusual methods of treatment and your fee schedule. Talking about the staff and patients is okay. Talk about the demographics of the area and all the positive things that are happening nearby. Show them the office and any special equipment, etc. You can talk about why you are selling and your post-sale plans, but limit the first meeting to these topics.

DO: Always be positive and considerate of the buyer candidate. In most cases this is the first time the buyer will be going through a purchase. They may seem nervous or anxious but this is normal as they are young and have never experienced anything like this before. Unfortunately, dental school does very little if any to prepare dentists for the transition process or practice ownership.

DO NOT: Show your tax returns or other practice financial information until you feel that the candidate is interested.

DO NOT: Discuss the terms of the sale, purchase price, lower down payment, the number of years, etc. There is no need for these discussions in the first meeting.

DO NOT: Allow the purchaser candidate to review your records; there is no reason to do so until following the first meeting.

DO NOT: Allow the buyer candidate to get a copy of your patient list.

DO NOT: Let the purchaser candidate make copies of your records, access your computer, or call any of your patients or referral sources.

DO NOT: Talk to the purchaser's attorney or accountant. This is better handled by a professional that has experience in dealing with these advisors.

DO NOT: Agree to anything to which you are uncertain; check with your advisor first.

DO NOT: "Badmouth" the competition, but also don't build them up too much either!

Just remember what you were like when you were the same age and be prepared to be a little forgiving. A new dentist will either (I) believe that he/she is smarter and is a better dentist than you; or (II) be scared to death to decide; or (III) if you are fortunate, confident but appreciative of the opportunity. Remember, you are probably too old to know everything, but he or she is not!

So, what makes up a successful transition? Dental transitions happen all over the country with and without practice brokers. So how does one complete a successful transition? Completing a transition doesn't make it a success. In fact, I have countless stories of doctors I've heard of buying or selling practices on their own that ended up being complete failures for them or the other party involved. I'd be willing to bet that you've heard these stories from some of your friends or colleagues. So why do dentists continue to allow this to happen. In most cases dentists have the persona of the "do it yourself" mentality. This can be great clinically as it will allow you to dive into a lot more procedures than you might have expected when graduating dental school. Unfortunately, this attitude doesn't translate well when it comes time to run a practice or transition. There are many components to a successful transition but the easiest way to phrase it is a WIN-WIN for both parties. For it to be a win-win both party's needs & goals need to be met with the sale and acquisition.

Potential purchasers answering classified ads of this kind are looking for a "deal." They want to "negotiate" and drive a hard bargain. Even if the practice is already underpriced, they want to pay less. Answering phone calls that interrupt your schedule during the day and evenings, disclosing confidential information to unqualified buyers, losing staff and patients troubled by an uncertain future are but a few of the "rewards" for the doctor attempting to sell his or her practice. You could also find yourself paying legal, and accounting fees for incomplete transactions carried out in the typical adversarial selling environment.

Then, we have the discount practice brokers who begin the relationship by offering a "deal." They are going to sell your practice and charge you a lower fee. Of course, everyone knows the value of his or her service, and if you pay less, you must be willing to accept less. Accepting less means less comprehensive appraisals, no computerized income and expense proformas, no pre-screening or qualifying buyer candidates, no contracts or worse, inadequate agreements that leave the door open to post-sale litigation. Add this to a negotiated selling price, and the seller is going to lose an awful lot of money because he/she focused more on the seller fee than the practice sale price.

Discount brokers make up in volume what they don't make on each transaction. How? They do this by undervaluing the practice with hopes that it will sell quickly. By trying to save money on the commission, the seller can lose tens of thousands of dollars by accepting a below market purchase price for the practice. There is no such thing as a free lunch. A discounted commission means a less comprehensive service and a lower selling price.

At AFTCO, we help dentists by focusing on what will give the seller and buyer the greatest result from a transition. Positioning your practice correctly for a future sale will result in you getting top dollar for your practice which in turn will give the buyer the greatest opportunity for success. If the buyer is successful, he/she will be able to care much more for your patients and staff. To learn how to position your practice for a future transition visit www.aftco.net or call 480-634-4803.

Chapter 7

Interview with Dr. Bob Shelton

For those of you who don't know Dr. Bob Shelton, he is a retired dentist in Tucson that graduated from the University of Minnesota in 1965. He had a successful career lasting until 2011 when he retired from clinical dentistry. Since then he has assisted and consulted with many dentists in Tucson and the surrounding areas. Given his story we decided to interview him for your benefit to hear the process from one of your colleague's perspective. As luck would have it he agreed as he has been through the process and hopes it will help all the dentists considering a change in the near future. He understands the emotional and psychological stress it can have when it is done incorrectly and then the joy it can bring when done correctly.

Please enjoy the interview below as I believe it will give you the perspective you're looking for from an experienced dentist who has gone through the process before in the not too distant past.

Chad: All right, Bob. Can you please start with your history in dentistry?

Bob: I started my own practice in 1979 in Tucson. Then moved to a different location, bought a practice in the early 90's and worked there for "X" number of years. I had an associate at the time with the intention to create a partnership. In other words, he buys in for half and then when I retire, he would buy the second half. It became apparent quickly that he wouldn't want to do that because he built up his practice within my practice to the point that he didn't need the second half. We became 50-50 partners and he did buy in for 50%. Then, it became obvious that neither one of us wanted to necessarily be paying profit sharing and so forth, mostly because of tax reasons. I was quite a bit older than this guy. We dissolved that partnership and he moved a year or two later up the street to build his own building. Now, I got my practice back and re-sold it.

During the transition with Todd, way before AFTCO, we went through a very tough time trying to transition the office. I've said this before, but the one big mistake that dentists make is thinking that they can do this on their own and thinking they're smart enough to do so because they're dentists. We went through CPA's and lawyers and put together agreements that never came. Then, when I was ready to think about selling, I contacted AFTCO. That's when we met Tim and talked with him before we listed.

I didn't want to retire; nor could I afford to retire at that point. We found buyers named Luis and Katrina. They purchased the practice and I continued to work. We did a pre-sale in the classic AFTCO sense. It worked great. I worked for two and half, maybe three years as a provider for them. Then, I decided to stop working at that point. It was a pre-sale with an open-ended work contract, so that I could work if I wanted to.

Chad: You're telling a great story, but if I'm a dentist I'm thinking: "You did a pre-sale and you continued working there. What was it that Tim said that convinced you that a pre-sale makes sense?" If I were a dentist without all this knowledge, I would be thinking "Well, my best bet is that I should stay in as an owner for as long as possible because I'm going to have more profit. Then, at the very end when I'm ready to retire, that's when I'm going to pull the trigger and just sell my practice." I would guess that's probably what most dentists are thinking. What was it that convinced you that maybe that's not the best move?

Bob: I think most dentists do think that way. One, I was probably older than the average dentist who decides to sell. I was 65 and didn't have enough money to retire. Maybe it was with Tim's advice. I didn't know what a pre-sale was. I said to Tim, "Well, I don't know if I'm really ready to sell." He educated me that you don't have to sell and leave the practice altogether.

It was at the peak at my productivity. Looking at the big picture I said, "Well, I certainly don't want to be selling and listing a declining practice." I wasn't worn out and tired. I was down to three days a week toward the end and still productive. So, I was still at the height of my productivity. I realized after advice from Tim that I could take this great asset and use that money to help fund my plan, but still make an income for a while.

Chad: Did it resonate with you that, "Gosh, I'm at my peak of productivity now. I'm down to three days, but in another few years I could make more money." Was that going through your mind at all?

Bob: Yeah. I didn't want to work harder. We even talked along the way even before that about growing the practice and addressed the issue of marketing. My style of practice was that we really didn't need any more new patients. I was maxed out in my head. I didn't want to work harder or longer hours. We had, I don't know, twenty new patients a month. That was maxed out to me.

Chad: You feel like that's a message that could resonate with most dentists?

Bob: Yeah. I would say that it does. We've had that conversation with a lot of dentists who are 58. They say, "Well, I'm going to really build this up. I'm 3 to 5 years away." How long have you heard that conversation?

Chad: Yeah. (laughs)

Bob: If we could make them look at doing it now and show them the math for their own practice, then I know it would make sense. We did the math for mine and said "Well, if we can get this 70 - 80% value now, and still work and make, I don't know what I was making, a couple hundred thousand? As a provider, it's a no-brainer. Then we worked out the financing whereby I got 50% down. Then financed, I think it was 7% for 10 years, which was great for me and for my situation.

I got the lump sum and then was getting "X" thousand a month payment, while collecting "X" for being a provider, too. I was getting three sources of income.

Chad: Did you want to do that initially, though, or did you not want to do that? What was your first reaction to carrying that amount?

Bob: I wanted to do that because of the buyers. I knew them. I had great faith. I think that must be a huge trust issue. If you have a great relationship with the buyers, or get to know them personally, it helps. I guess not everyone can do that. There's big trust there.

Chad: How long before did you know him? Did you know him for a while, or just a short period?

Bob: Mary, my daughter, worked in my practice for 15 years. She also did some consulting for other practices they had worked in. Anyway, she does consulting for them and knew the buyers. They were the big producers down there because they did implants and prosth. The buyer, Luis, was looking for a practice to buy and Mary introduced us. There was a lot of trust up front even before Tim met them as well. That was a little unique to have that kind of introduction made and build that quick of a relationship with the buyer.

Chad: That is unique.

Bob: I still love the process. There's trust and due diligence with AFTCO and when it's done that way, yeah, the pre-sale with the carry back I liked a lot.

Chad: So, you were 65 and you decided that now is the time that you were going to start looking at making a change. Did you contact us directly? How much searching did you do to find the right consultant, and when you found them how did you know that was the right fit?

Bob: I knew about you both because of a friend of mine. I didn't tell you that story. The doctor who I bought the practice from originally had spoken with you in the past. After I had this somewhat disastrous "trying-to-do it-on-our-own" with lawyers and CPA's paying big money, and not getting great results, I knew about you both so I called immediately.

Chad: What kind of emotions were you feeling when you decided it was time to make a change? Were all the emotions of your practice gone and you just said I need retirement, or what did you feel along the way from the minute that you were considering making a change to the time when you were working with Tim? Then afterwards, what kind of emotional roller coaster did you go through?

Bob: I would say not a big roller coaster for me at all.

Chad: Okay.

Bob: We knew the "trying-to-do it-on-our-own" was a roller coaster because there's a lot of negatives and that's not going to work. We had to re-write and take it to a different lawyer and that kind of game they play. Nancy and I, my wife of 53 years, had 17 houses and 18 RV's. That tells you that I'm not that attached to material things or even businesses. We knew it was an asset that at some point needed to be sold and the money taken out of it. We did the math.

Chad: It wasn't as super emotional in your case. I think a lot of times dentists are tied emotionally to their patients.

Bob: Oh! I have a friend just like that. He's got these patients he cares deeply about and vice versa. He worries about keeping his staff, too. I had that, but I just knew the big picture was if we found the right buyer, and I could continue to work, and we did the math and that, I had "X" dollars that I could use to fund my retirement—this is what needed to be done. In other words, once I saw on paper that this would work financially and we had the right buyer, then it wasn't emotional. It was just a done deal in my head.

Same when I retired and quit. I think it was maybe two and a half years as a provider, and six months before my 68th birthday, I said one morning to my wife, "I'm going to retire on my birthday. I'm uninspired." I'd never, ever felt that way about dentistry. I always loved getting up in the morning going to work. The staff, the patients; I loved that whole thing until 6 months before.

Chad: Interesting.

Bob: It was very sudden. The buyers were in place. I was working two, two and a half days by then. I said, "That's it, I'm done on my 68th birthday." I think dentists know that in their heart of hearts if they can be shown that they can make this work financially, if they are shown the numbers whether it's pre-sale or walk away or however that's structured, then it's worth doing. It's like people buying a house. If the great consultants create a situation where that person can see themselves in that house, dentists can see himself or herself going through with a transition. They say, "Oh yeah, I think I can see myself doing that— buying a motorhome or driving off into the sunset." They must see the possible before it's probable.

Chad: After you went to work with the buyer and you gave up control to him and he owned the practice, what was your experience like? Do you have any regrets from that? Was it all positive? What did you like and not like about it?

Bob: I loved that because they were young and inexperienced and I was a bit of a mentor. That was a real positive. With staff, staff meetings, conflict resolution—I could be the mentor. Then, I loved that part too because I was a father figure to these young women with personal problems and the whole thing in any organization. I loved that part. I think I mentored them a bit.

There was only one conflict that I can remember that ever came up with the buyers and myself, and that was had to do with the hygienist seeing the new patient and doing the perio probing and charting. Katrina wanted the doctors to do the perio probing and charting and I was adamant that the hygienist needed to do that. We got into a debate about that. I said, "Well, you're taking her power away; that's her job and that's what she's trained to do. You need to establish that association and that relationship with that patient up front was my point. How do you hand off to the hygienist who's never seen that patient, but you've done all the perio charting and educating, and blah, blah, blah?" That was the only conflict. They did it my way when all was said and done.

Otherwise, they're great managers. Mary, my daughter, still works for them to this day. They were mature, though, and that was a huge help.

Chad: So, you're technically an independent contractor or employee after the sale. What would have happened if she would have said, "No. I think you're wrong," or "I want to do it my way." Would that have been a real tough pill for you to swallow?

Bob: Personally, but I would have. If in any point in time she were that strong about it, I would've said, "Hey, you guys own this practice and I'll back off. I just want you to know that I feel strongly that the hygienist needs to perform this service." I would have backed off for sure.

Chad: I'm trying to picture dentists that own their own practice for 25 years and now some young dentist comes in and is dictating, saying, "We need to do it this way." How long did it take for that to sink in? Maybe it was just that you had another negative experience before, maybe it just made sense right from the get go to present that?

Bob: I think my nature is to trust unless that's betrayed. Then, I'm your worst enemy. So, I trust the first time. It was a betrayal in a way with the first transition. It was such a terrible experience and I decided to trust the new buyer and you guys to know what you're doing. It was wonderful. I was never suspicious of the process or anything like that.

Chad: Your unique position is that you did go through two very different scenarios; whereas, most doctors, like we've talk about, they're out 30 or 40 years practicing. They get one chance to sell their practice. You had an adversarial transition that didn't go through and then you had one that was on dual representation. Comparing the two, would you ever go back to any type of adversarial transition on a dental practice related transition? Is there any reason that you would ever consider using that form instead of dual representation?

Bob: No, it just works...you guys have been in Arizona for over 30 years and have completed significantly more transitions than anyone else. There's got to be something good about that.

Chad: Right. What was your favorite thing that you liked about the dual representation model where we work with the buyer and the seller throughout the process?

Bob: I think the fair representation and the fair education of both buyer and seller. Tim met with the buyers separately and then together. We did a normal due diligence process. It always seemed equal with Tim. He worked with them and he worked with me. It was an open book. We weren't telling secrets either way. That was some of it. I can't think of negatives at all. It's unique. Is there anyone else out in the market selling practices in this fashion?

Chad: No. They typically represent the seller. I don't know of anyone here in Arizona that use dual representation. It is certainly unique.

Bob: I think it's probably common and inviting to a dentist
      when a typical broker salesman comes in and says,
      "Hey, I think I can get you $700,000 for your practice."
      That's kind of inviting.

Chad: That's an incentive there?

Bob: Yeah, but it's strictly money. They don't realize that
      there's a lot more to it than just that.

Chad: Yes, absolutely.

Bob: The thing Tim used a lot is, "Your job as the buyer is to
      make the seller happy, and your job as the seller is to
      make the buyer happy."

Chad: Now that you're past the sale of your practice is there
      anything that you know now that you wish you knew
      back then when you were transitioning your practice?

Bob: Yeah, I would've called Tim about five years earlier.

Chad: Was there any part of the process, as far as
      education that was given and the way the transition
      was handled? Is there any point where you wish you
      would've known more or that Tim would've touched on
      a few more items to give you more clarity throughout
      the process or was it evenly step by step, walking you,
      kind of holding your hand throughout the process to
      make sure that it got handled smoothly?

Bob: I just have overall good feelings about the whole
      transition. Tim handled everything from start to finish
      and made it a very seamless process. I think that's the
      trust issue thing I talked about earlier though— not
      wanting to read that contract; I'd rather watch paint dry.
      I was bored with all of that. It was way too technical for

me. I remember internally saying, "I'm glad you know what you're doing." I'm old and out of touch with the details. I was a detailed dentist, but I'm not a detailed business person. I remember looking at the contract thinking, "When's this day going to end?" I'm bored by that stuff and I trust that someone knows what they're doing. At least subconsciously, I was thinking that, "Why do I have to go through all this because it's been done 10,000 other times." Some dentists are like engineer types. If we had a dental patient who was an engineer, he's got one of those pocket protectors, and the first question they ask is, "How many RPM's is that air turbine?"

Chad: Did they really ask you that?

Bob: Yes. I had a guy, he's a professional engineer, ask me that once. I said, "Well, this one goes about 400,000 RPM." He said, "That's impossible. It would fall apart." He starts arguing with me about RPM. That's the engineer mindset or even, "What's the percentage of gold in that crown?" That kind of talk. Those people would read every line of a contract. I think knowing the personality of the dentist will help decide which type of buyer is best for their practice.

Chad: So, fast forward to today since you're mostly retired. With most older doctors, I hear one word more often than any others. That word is "fear". They get to the point that they've been doing dentistry for so long that they realize that's all that they know and all that they do. They lose their hobbies. Their kids are grown. They're out. They're empty nesters. A lot of the doctors that I've talked to, fear retirement. They fear that change, if you will. Right now, they at least know the practice might not be doing well. They might have problems and issues, but at least they know those problems and issues. They know what that is. They've got that level of comfort of knowing day in and day out what they're going to be expecting. Most doctors, if that's the case, they tend to fear that retirement.

Do you have any suggestions for them? Did you fear retirement at that point? How are you liking retirement? Kind of expand a little on that that might help them feel a little better about making that move.

Bob: You're good at that in the meetings. I've been with you in meetings too, I guess you can call it "education," but it's really "questions," in that initial meeting. We begin to educate..."What kind of things do you like to do? What kind of hobbies?" We can see that there's some interests to touch on and then translate that to, "Well, you're going to have a hell of a lot more time now to go RV'ing, or to go sailing, or travel to Europe or whatever it is that they have in here that they haven't been able to do.

The ones who have forgotten their hobbies, I think would love it again. I think the answer to your question is that I think we need to find out up front if we can simulate interests in them to make them realize there's a whole world out there before drilling teeth. I mean, other than drilling holes in teeth. I don't know if that's the answer, but I think we need to find the interests out first and then educate or motivate, if you will. I think the message here is: "there is life after dentistry."

Chad: Exactly. I think the message there is that the hobbies that they don't do now could be because dentistry gets in the way. It could be that when they get out, even after you've got done with dentistry and you've decided, "Okay, I'm now 68 and I'm retiring," You didn't immediately go and sit on your porch and hock bottles at kids for running across your lawn. You didn't play the grumpy old man. You went out and you're RV'ing around now. You're playing pickleball and golf— the things that you like to do.

Bob: I think we probably need to show that there can be an "Aha!" experience. Let's crunch some numbers and just see if this is do-able kind of mentality. Tim point blank asked one of our more entrepreneurial guys, "What's your financial goal? What do you need?" He said, "$17 million." Well, me personally, I don't need $17 million and that's different for everybody. For me, that's an illusion.

It's like when they interviewed T. Boone Pickens, the Texas multi-billionaire, that oil guy. In his early 80's, he was putting in pipeline to Dallas from Northern Texas and he had underground rights to minerals, so he had Wind Farms and multi-billion-dollar piping water to Dallas. The interviewer, it might have been on *60 Minutes*, says, "Well, Mr. Pickens, obviously, you don't need the money, but how much money do you need?" Pickens kind of went like this, "just a little bit more."

Chad: Like Tom Brady: "Which super bowl ring is your favorite?" and his answer, "the next one."

Bob: It's like that. It's an illusion. Can you live on a couple million dollars? That sounds impossible to a young dentist who owes $400,000. If you can show them with the math that at some point in time they can do this, it's the "Aha!" You can fund your retirement plans with the assets and then still work. You can have the best of both worlds.

Chad: It's fun to get these dentists to see the vision. They're so overwhelmed with their $400,000 - $600,000 worth of student loans and they can't even imagine having $2,000,000, so they just as well might imagine having $100,000,000. They can't envision that. It's so far gone to be able to make that real. It's good to hear you confirm that it's important.

Bob: Yeah, that initial meeting and questions ignite answers for them that they would never ask themselves.

Chad: Plant seeds even.

Bob: Yes. It is seed planting. Their pupils dilate, "Wow, I can actually accomplish my goals using dentistry as the vehicle to get me there."

Chad: Would you would have enjoyed that early in your career? Having somebody help guide you through the process and goal set?

Bob: Dentistry is overwhelming when you think about everything that goes into it, as well as the home life it creates. I was at retirement thinking, "Man, this is stressful." Making a living for your family and the work is stressful. Financially it's demanding. You don't want to come across desperate to a patient, like "I need the money, so you should do this bridge." You got to be a psychologist, a boss, a financial planner, etc.

Chad: It really is. I guess for the dentist you are really saying that, but that's our role as well.

Bob: I think you hit on something Chad. You must educate at their level. We teach" "pickleball." I don't know if you know what "pickleball" is? We teach "pickleball" to old people who are beginners. You can see these "Aha!" moments, but the teaching...It's hard to be a teacher when you know a lot about something, because you can overwhelm them and give them way too many details. Where are they at this level?" They're not professional "pickleball" players. How do I teach at

75

their level? How do you teach, like you said, the kid who is half a million in debt and can't see his way to climbing out of that hole? How do we teach at that level? I think the neat thing we need to say to the younger dentist is, "You're doing the work. I'm the teacher here, but you got to do the hard work. You just got to do a little nose to the grindstone for the next 15 years and you're only 30. You can do this. You can see your way. They must see their way clear as young buyers.

Chad: Let me ask you a couple questions because these young buyers. Some of these practices that we have where the margins are just phenomenal. We could put a young dentist into Gilbert and maybe make $125,000. We can put him in Sierra Vista and make half a million to a million. For me, it's a no brainer. What is it about, and I'm generalizing here big time, what is it about these young dentists that so few of them are willing to go rural? Is it something that happens in dental school?

Bob: Not sure. That's a good one to explore. You would think a young dentist who's married or even married with a family already, wouldn't be wanting to go to nightclubs and night stuff like that like they do in Phoenix. I know that's a big reason why young people would rather live in Phoenix than Tucson. There's more action up here. More stuff, right?

Chad: More ways to get in trouble than you know it.

Bob: Yeah. Nothing good happens after 2AM.

Chad: Not only that. In these bigger cities, there's so many dentists that it almost cheapens the value. Not a dime a dozen, but you know what I'm saying. You're a pillar of community.

76

Bob: Absolutely.

Chad: Does that resonate with you? If you're a young dentist coming out of school and you can get into an opportunity where you can pay off your loans in just a few short years, as well as create the financial stability you always dreamed of, are those things that are important to you? Do you care what your community thinks about you?

Bob: I do. In other words, the big fish in the little pond kind of thinking; although, it's not really.

Chad: That's been maybe the most frustrating thing for me, since I've been here. I just don't understand. It seems like they ought to be tripping over themselves to get to these other practices that are less expensive to maintain because they make more money and there's a lot less competition.

Bob: I don't think that's a bad thing to say what you just said. "Young doc, tell me something. I'm just curious about this. Look at the numbers here. In my way of thinking, why wouldn't you trip over yourself to get into this practice? You could make $300,000 - $500,000 the first year you're there. Why wouldn't you do that. I'm just curious about what is it that holds you back from doing that? That's an unbelievable opportunity."

Chad: I think that when they're in dental school a lot of doctors that come out kind of have a false sense of confidence. Not just on a clinical level, but on the business level as well. The typical thinking is, "I can go anywhere in the country and I'll be successful." If they look at their predecessors before them, their dads that were dentists or their grandfathers that were dentists, it was kind of that way for them 20-40 years ago.

I think that the last 10 years have defined dentistry and what it will be in the future. Bob, even back when you had your practice, what worked back in 1991 wouldn't work in today's market. I'm sure you'd agree today that the community and everything involved is very different.

The way to build your practice today is very different than it was back then. It was more that the individual could build the practice, but now there's a lot more outside circumstances that are controlling that. Almost every doctor I talk to, they say, "Well, that's not me. I'm the exception." It seems like that's always the excuse I get is, "Oh, well, I'm not going to be like those dentists. I'm not going to do it like that dentist. I'm not going to do those things. I'm smart. I'm too smart to do that."

Bob: When I got out of school I just knew it would work. I just knew how to make it work. In today's world, I would be thinking a lot differently, though. There are a lot of new factors constantly entering the market and if the doctor doesn't know how to handle them they can quickly get buried. It's all about learning to be responsive and not reactive.

Bob: I don't know if it was Mandela, or some famous, influential person, said something like, "People aren't as afraid of failure as they are of wild success, because it takes on..." You know that quote? It takes on new responsibility." If I get this successful, wow, that means I must be the pillar of the community and perform.

Chad: That's interesting.

Bob: There's much more pressure on wild success than failure.

Chad: That makes a lot of sense. Think about the amount of change that you had to have to become wildly successful; not just internally, but around you, and what you would have to change within yourself to get there. Whereas failure, you can fail as the person that you are today. You're not out of your comfort zone. You don't ever step out of your comfort zone to fail.

Bob: I could even do less.

Chad: That's right.

Chad: I'm seeing these young dentists and they're a little bit nervous and there is a sense of peace and relief just going to work for one of these corporate places. It's not where I wanted to be but it's okay. I can just go there and they'll provide the patients for me and I get my daily guarantee. So, they're just settling.

Bob: An old friend and I were just talking about this last night. We're old dental school classmates. We're both 75 and we're talking about millennials and generation X. Especially millennials. The perception we have, us old people have, is that they are taught to be special. Our 14-year-old granddaughter was in a gymnastics meet and the ceremony for giving out ribbons lasted longer than the gymnastics meet itself. She got a 14th place overall ribbon. Now, fast forward that generation to being in the workforce and all they've been told is, you're very special, you get special treat for graduating or just showing up. They have graduation ceremonies for kindergarten nowadays and then they hit the real world later in life and I think that's the generation you're seeing and why they're nervous. "Holy crap, I don't know how to do this. I was always given everything and I was told I was so special and so wonderful." Where in the old days, it was almost the opposite.

Chad: That's usually what I see the first year or two out there that way where they come out thinking the same thing. Thinking they're special and that they're entitled to making a ton of money, or they're going to do much better than everyone else around them. Then the market beats them up a little and suddenly, they realize that they bleed just like everybody else and that's when they find out that they're going to have to buckle down to create any type of success. If you can find a doctor that's been out for two years and on, you have much better rate of selling them your practice or transitioning them into a partnership.

Bob: Some dentists, I think that we work with, are learning all there is to know about dentistry in four years of dental school and repeating that forty years in a row. I think that happens. They get stifled, or plateau, or however you want to say that. And the young guy, the really young guys, first week he's working he has an employee, say a young woman, and she comes in and says, "I need a raise." They don't know how to deal with that stuff and I think that's where they get nervous.

Chad: What about the doctors that are considering going to work for public health?

Bob: Yeah.

Chad: And they'll give part of their student loans taken care of, so that seems to be popular and fashionable and something they wanted to do but we haven't had the same amount of luck convincing them to buy a practice where, forget about them paying for it. Look how much, you can pay off your own loans if we can get you this practice. Because when you go there, yeah, they're paying off a portion of your debt but you're making considerably less.

Bob: It might be the assuredness of the saying that a bird in the hand is worth two in the bush. It might be that. They get comfortable and unfortunately, that is the #1 killer of dreams!

Chad: Is there any other advice that you would give? Anything else that you would tell dentists that reach 55 and over? Or some advice to dentists whose practices plateaued? What do you think they ought to be considering at that point?

Bob: One of the first things out of their mouth when I contact a dentist, and I've contacted maybe three, four, five in the last month, is: "Well, I'm not ready to sell yet." So, they're very narrowly focused early on, and only want to discuss anything when they are ready to actually do it. We can't get our foot in the door with that mentality. I'm not sure you can do this on the phone, but they need to see the possibilities. I think somehow, we should get a meeting with them to show that there are other possibilities out there, and waiting until you are in the mood or feel like you're "ready" to sell your practice, isn't smart. I don't think we're ever ready, financially or emotionally. It's an illusion to think that way. If I could instill just one thing with every doctor I know, is to figure out your options years before you need to exercise them.

This is a huge help when planning your retirement, as well as ensuring your family is taken care of if something happens to you. This goes for old and young dentists. I transitioned my practice with Chad and Tim and it could not have gone any better. If you don't have a clear-cut plan for the next 10 years I highly recommend setting a meeting and getting something hammered out before it turns to regret.

Bob could reach a successful transition due to careful planning and working with AFTCO to create a win-win transition. This resulted in him achieving his retirement goals, while still being able to practice clinically even after he sold. This allowed him to travel as much as he liked while phasing out of clinical dentistry. To make your own dreams a reality, call 480-634-4803 or visit www.aftco.net.

Testimonials
Practice Transition Done the Right Way

Dr. Agnew

You know you can't work like this forever. Whether you are at the daydream phase or the decision point, you owe it to yourself to evaluate your options. Life's next great adventure lurks around the corner.

After 30 years of loving my work, my patients and my lifestyle, I knew it was time to get after that bucket list. Like you, I attended those retirement seminars only to feel the practice transition companies had business models that just did not fit my practice realities or my retirement vision.

Then I meet Chad Flake, Transition Analyst for AFTCO. Chad is extremely dynamic and intelligent, and most importantly an energetic listener! He focused on my practice style and personal requirements, envisioning my perfect transition and then bringing it to fruition. Experienced, personable and dedicated, he found the optimal practitioner to continue my labor of love. The transition was philosophically, financially and emotionally ideal for me, the buyer and so importantly, my beloved patients. It was, as is said, a match made in heaven.

Chad and his AFTCO team worked diligently making sure all the details were properly addressed. He was always only a phone call away. Difficulties presented only as opportunities to excel and better the transition. The transition has been a seamless success for all. I attribute this exceptional outcome directly to Chad and AFTCO. He listened to my needs and expectations, and found the consummate professional to continue my practice to the delight of my patients.

While I am busy following new dreams, I remain forever grateful to Chad for getting me here. I strongly recommend Chad Flake of AFTCO for your practice transition. Do it the right way with outstanding success and no regrets. I would love to discuss my transition process with anyone.   Please contact me directly should I be of any assistance to you in your practice transition journey.

Best Regards,
Beverly R Agnew, DDS

Dr. Rosenthal

I am a 63-year-old dentist that was ready for a change. I have been a dentist for 37 years and had been in the same location for 27 years. Due to personal issues, I was ready to walk away from my practice. I just wanted to get out alive! Out of desperation I called AFTCO and was connected with

Chad Flake. Chad carefully listened to my desires and wants and over the next two weeks came up with an exit strategy that would allow me

to keep practicing dentistry without all the headaches and to leave with my dignity intact. Chad found a buyer that bought my practice and then merged my entire staff and patients into another practice that had the latest in dental technology.

I was amazed at how smoothly the transition went! Chad and his team carefully led me through the merger, step by step; and there were a lot of steps. I never had to figure anything out. Chad kept me abreast of what was happening daily either with phone calls or via e-mail. The excellent communication was greatly appreciated on my end.

The entire process from when I first met Chad to doing dentistry in another location took six weeks. I couldn't be happier. I work three days a week
taking care of my old patients in a beautiful facility. The best part is I am just doing dentistry and no longer have to run the business.

I would highly recommend contacting Chad Flake to discuss a future exit strategy. There are many possibilities. It is much better to have this discussion sooner than later!

Dr. Howard

I am writing to share my experience with Chad Flake. I had tried to either sell or transition my practice with the help of other transition experts and was unsuccessful. AFTCO" s expertise was evident from the first consultation. They represented both the buyer and the seller and both parties were very pleased with the outcome. Their appraisal brought interested dentists to my office and I could interview several people who shared with me their philosophy of treatment and their experience such that I could find the best person to continue the care of my patients. My staff was retained with the buyer so that the transition was smooth for my staff and him. The contract that was prepared was excellent and needed little revision. My CPA and I found that it was so well done that I did not contact an attorney to review it. I found that the transition did not interfere with my daily dental schedule. They even found a lender that would accept the agreement without underwriting problems. I would recommend AFTCO to any dentist that wants to have a smooth, rapid, equitable sale of his/ her practice.

Dr. Taylor

We have completed three successful practice purchases and transitions with Chad Flake. Chad is very knowledgeable and extremely helpful. He will always get back to you with an answer ASAP. Even after the deal is done, Chad will remain available. Chad's chief concerns are fitting you with the right practice and ensuring the most successful transition.

Mr. McGee

Overall it was a great experience. Chad was very knowledgeable about the process from start to finish. He also put us in contact with people to help us move the process along. The due diligence that was given to us for the practice we purchased allowed us to analyze and make the decision of purchasing much easier. We look forward to working with Chad and AFTCO again in the future.

Dr. LaVant

Chad Flake was very personal and attentive to the needs and negations of both parties. He was very instrumental in the process, I had a lot of questions in which he took his time to answer or if he did not know the answer would get back in contact with me very quickly after he found out. I would recommend working with Chad. My first impression of Chad was that he looked very young and he was just another broker trying to make a sale, that was not the case at all, he is very knowledgeable and guided me through the transition process better than some of these brokers who have way more years in the field. Thank you very much Chad and I look forward to working with you again and buying more practices.

Dr. Crawford

Chad: I want to thank you for a smooth transition of my practice here in Tucson. You were very attentive and answered all my questions as we went to the process. I recommend you and your company for my teacher friends. Thank you!

Author Biographies

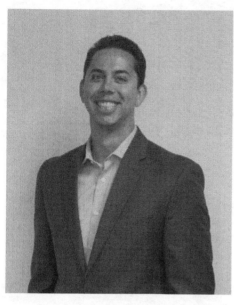

Chad Flake
Senior Regional Transition Analyst

None of you reading this were born a dentist and none of you need to die a dentist if you follow our tested and proven system. Our doctors enjoy a happier more successful lifestyle with more free time to spend with family, friends, and doing other activities they might enjoy. What I'm talking about is creating the financial freedom to do what you want with who you want and all on your schedule when you want to do it. For many this can be a pipe dream due to poor planning and even worse, poor execution. Chad's vision and leadership has helped countless dentists reach the retirement they had always dreamed of!

You can't have Financial Freedom with poor planning and poor execution. Financial Freedom is given to those that have a strong plan and back that plan with MASSIVE action! Dentistry has only gotten tougher over the years and will continue to increase in difficulty as time progresses. There are threats from large DSO's, Insurance providers reducing fees, increasing number of graduating dentists creating more competition in markets across the country and so on and so forth. If you're a practicing dentist you've likely faced these issues already.

Chad is a Senior Regional Transition Analyst with AFTCO and has been transitioning dental practices and consulting with dentists for nearly a decade. He has been involved in hundreds of dental transitions ranging from sales, acquisitions, mergers, partnerships and many other detailed transitions. Throughout these transitions, he has also consulted with countless doctors to assist in growing their practices.

While Chad isn't working with dentists he is spending time with his three children (Courtney, Max and Abi) or in the desert off road racing.

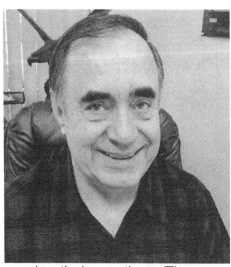

Tim Wildung
Regional Director
AFTCO

Tim Wildung began his career in dentistry in January 1989 when he met Alan Thornberg. Having had personal friends who were dentists and seeing the struggles his friends were having running their practices; Tim saw this as a great solution to these issues that seemed to beset his friends, which made this a natural for his next entrepreneurial venture. Prior to this, Tim owned and managed a securities firm specializing in tax shelters and financial planning. He has spent most of his life as an entrepreneur establishing and growing various ventures.

In 1995 after spending over 6 years consulting dentists he began Family Dental in the Arizona market wherein he purchased several practices. Growing the business to 8 practices by 1998, Family Dental and Dental One merged into one regional company covering AZ, TX, CO & UT. Continuing as V.P. of Operations, Tim and team grew the business to 55 practices by 2002.

These experiences give Tim a unique perspective to be one of the foremost experts in consulting and advising dentists on the business side of dentistry. He has helped numerous dentists achieve financial freedom and become financially secure. His main objective is to show dentists how to rise above the odds, as 96% of dentists cannot retire at the same economical level that they had while they were working. (ADA, 2016)

Made in the USA
San Bernardino, CA
25 May 2017